Contents

Reproduction authorization

The purchaser of this *Patient Pictures* series title is hereby authorized to reproduce by photocopy only, any part of the pictorial and textual material contained in this work for non-profit, educational, or patient education use. Photocopying for these purposes only is welcomed and free from further permission requirements from the publisher and free from any fee.

The reproduction of any material from this publication outside the guidelines above is strictly prohibited without the permission in writing of the publisher and is subject to minimum charges laid down by the Publishers Licensing Society Limited or its nominees.

Signed *Sarah Redston* Publisher, Health Press, Oxford

The publisher and the authors have made every effort to ensure the accuracy of this book, but cannot accept responsibility for any errors or omissions.

Cardiology

by
J Colin Forfar MD PhD FRCPE FRCP
Consultant Cardiologist, John Radcliffe Hospital,
and Honorary Senior Lecturer, University of Oxford, Oxford, UK

Series Editor
J Richard Smith MD MRCOG
Senior Lecturer and Honorary Consultant Gynaecologist,
Charing Cross and Westminster Medical School,
Chelsea and Westminster Hospital, London, UK

Illustrated by
Dee McLean, MeDee Art, London, UK

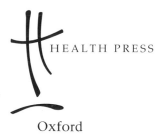

HEALTH PRESS

Oxford

Patient Pictures – Cardiology

First Published 1995

Reprinted 1997

© 1995 Health Press

Elizabeth House, Queen Street, Abingdon, Oxford OX14 3JR

A CIP catalogue record for this title is available from the British Library.

ISBN 1-899541-20-9

Managing editor: Amanda Klyne
Typeset by Impressions Design & DTP, Bicester, UK
Designed by Design Online, Oxford, UK
Printed by Uniskill, Witney, UK

Author's preface

Heart disease, sadly, remains a major killer in the western world.
Many heart conditions are, however, benign, and simply require
assessment and reassurance.

Over the past 20 years, exciting developments in the treatment and
prevention of heart disease have greatly improved the outlook for
heart patients. This has, however, meant that the assessment and
management of many different heart conditions often involves a
bewildering array of tests, complex investigations and treatments.

This book is designed to help to explain and increase understanding
of some of the more common heart disorders, and the procedures and
the treatments that are used.

I hope these words and pictures will facilitate the process of
communication between doctor and patient, and thereby reduce
some of the understandable anxieties that arise from a fear of the
unknown.

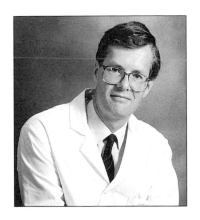

J Colin Forfar MD PhD FRCPE FRCP
Consultant Cardiologist
John Radcliffe Hospital
Oxford, UK

The heart and circulation

- The heart is a powerful muscular pump about the size of a fist that drives the circulation of blood to every part of the body. It beats about 100,000 times every 24 hours, or nearly 3 billion times in a lifetime. Depending on the body's needs, the heart can pump from 5 to 30 litres of blood per minute.

- The circulating blood takes oxygen from the lungs and energy-providing nutrients (fuel), such as fats and sugars from the liver, to all the body organs. It also carries away waste for removal; for example, carbon dioxide to the lungs, and waste nitrogen to the kidneys.

- Organs differ in the amount of oxygen and nutrients they need. For example, the kidneys and brain need plenty of oxygen to work normally, while the requirements of the muscles and gut depend on how active they are.

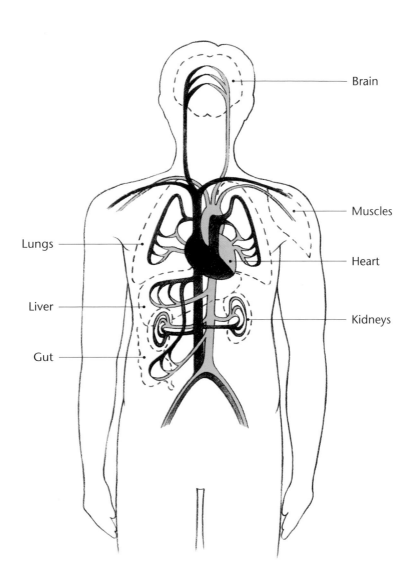

Brain

Muscles

Lungs

Heart

Liver

Kidneys

Gut

The heart as a pump

- The heart is actually two pumps in one. Each has a collecting chamber (atrium) above, a pumping chamber (ventricle) below, and one-way valves that prevent backflow.

- Blood carrying oxygen (red) from the lungs enters the left atrium through the four pulmonary veins and passes through the mitral valve into the powerful left ventricle which contracts, pumping it at high pressure to the body through the aortic valve, aorta and other arteries.

- Blood depleted of oxygen (blue) returns from the body through two large veins, the superior and inferior vena cavae, into the right atrium and passes through the tricuspid valve into the right ventricle, which is adapted to receive variable volumes of blood. The right ventricle pumps the deoxygenated blood to the lungs through the pulmonary valve and pulmonary arteries.

- For the heart to perform normally, it must pump vigorously, the valves must be intact, and the left ventricle must relax properly to receive blood from the left atrium.

- There are two phases to the heart pumping cycle – diastole and systole. Diastole is the period between contractions, when the muscle of the heart relaxes and the chambers fill with blood. Systole is the period during which the heart contracts.

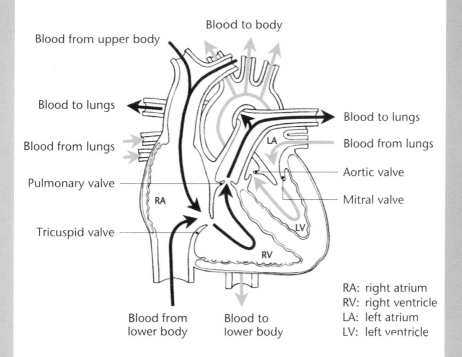

Blood to body

Blood from upper body

Blood to lungs

Blood from lungs

Pulmonary valve

Tricuspid valve

RA

LA

Blood to lungs

Blood from lungs

Aortic valve

Mitral valve

LV

RV

Blood from lower body

Blood to lower body

RA: right atrium
RV: right ventricle
LA: left atrium
LV: left ventricle

Blood carrying oxygen
Blood depleted of oxygen

HEART PUMPING CYCLE

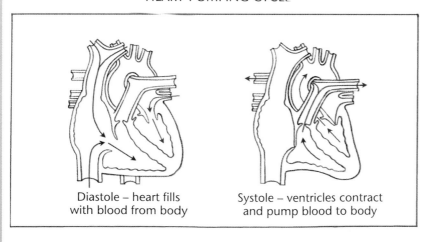

Diastole – heart fills with blood from body

Systole – ventricles contract and pump blood to body

The blood supply to the heart – the coronary arteries

- The heart circulates blood to every part of the body and must itself receive enough oxygenated blood to function properly. It uses about 10% of the body's oxygen needs at rest and more during exercise.

- Blood is supplied to the heart through the encircling coronary arteries. The two main coronary arteries, left and right, originate from the aorta, just above the aortic valve.

- The left main coronary artery splits into the circumflex branch, which supplies the back of the left ventricle, and the anterior descending branch, which supplies most of the rest of the left ventricle and the muscular wall between the right and left ventricles (interventricular septum).

- The right ventricle is supplied largely by the right coronary artery, which in most people also supplies part of the underside of the heart and part of the left ventricle. In about one-fifth of people, however, the right coronary artery is much smaller and the circumflex artery supplies the underside of the heart instead.

- Artery walls have three layers. The inner layer (endothelium) provides a slippery surface, which allows the blood to flow smoothly and minimizes blood clotting. The middle layer is strong, elastic and muscular; while the outer fibrous layer (adventitia) adds strength and contains tiny blood vessels that supply blood to the arteries themselves.

- Narrowing or obstruction of the coronary arteries is the main cause of a group of related disorders known as ischaemic heart disease (ischaemia means restriction in blood supply).

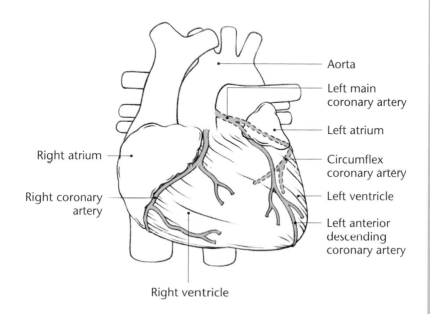

Aorta

Left main coronary artery

Left atrium

Circumflex coronary artery

Left ventricle

Left anterior descending coronary artery

Right atrium

Right coronary artery

Right ventricle

STRUCTURE OF THE CORONARY ARTERIES

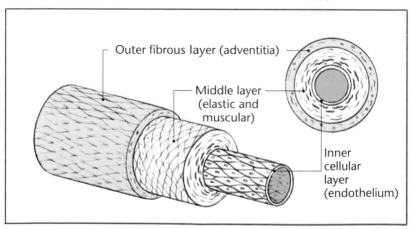

Outer fibrous layer (adventitia)

Middle layer (elastic and muscular)

Inner cellular layer (endothelium)

The heart valves

- The heart has four one-way valves. Two valves prevent blood from leaking back into the collecting chambers (atria) when the ventricles contract (the mitral valve on the left and the tricuspid valve on the right). The other two valves at the outlet of each ventricle prevent leakage from the main arteries back into the ventricles as they fill (the aortic valve on the left and the pulmonary valve on the right).

- Disease of the valves can cause leakage (regurgitation) and narrowing (stenosis); the aortic and mitral valves are most commonly affected.

- Disorders of the three-cusped aortic valve leading to stenosis or regurgitation can result from congenital abnormalities, 'wear and tear', or infection (endocarditis).

- The mitral valve is more complex. It has two cusps, each of which is anchored by fibrous strands (chordae – the 'heartstrings') to two papillary muscles arising from the left ventricle. These prevent the valve from turning inside out.

- The pulmonary valve resembles the aortic valve; congenital pulmonary stenosis may need to be corrected by an operation. The tricuspid valve resembles the mitral valve; leakage often causes little trouble because it works at low pressure, sealing the right ventricle from the right atrium as blood is pumped to the lungs.

- Operations to open up stenotic valves include stretching by passing a balloon along a blood vessel and inflating it, or surgery. Diseased valves can be replaced with artificial valves, or natural ones from pigs or donors.

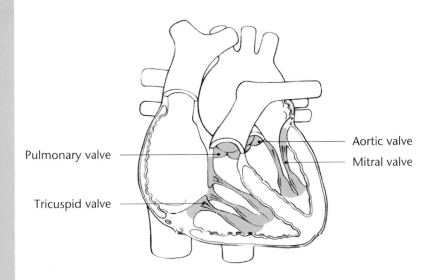

Pulmonary valve

Tricuspid valve

Aortic valve

Mitral valve

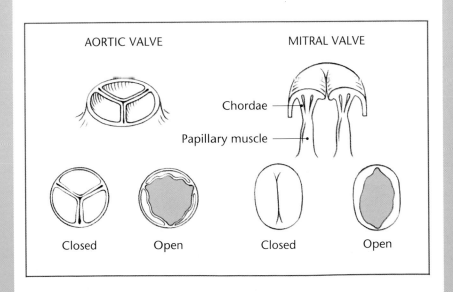

AORTIC VALVE

MITRAL VALVE

Chordae

Papillary muscle

Closed   Open   Closed   Open

Risk factors for heart disease

- Risk factors are aspects of a person's lifestyle, medical history or genetic make-up that increase their risk of suffering from a particular condition. Disease caused by disorders of the circulation to the heart is called coronary heart disease (CHD), and several risk factors for CHD are well known. Some are avoidable and/or treatable, while others are inherited.

- Smoking is the most important avoidable risk factor for CHD. Half of lifetime smokers die prematurely from their habit. You are two to five times more likely to die from a heart attack if you smoke than if you do not, but stopping smoking permanently cuts this risk considerably to little above that of a non-smoker after only a few years. It is never too late to stop!

- High blood pressure (hypertension) is a risk factor for stroke and heart attack that can easily be identified and treated.

- Other lifestyle risk factors for CHD include overeating leading to overweight, a high proportion of animal fats in the diet contributing to a high blood cholesterol, and lack of exercise.

- For complex reasons that are not well understood, early heart disease runs in families, so your risk of CHD is increased if young or middle-aged relatives are affected. Inherited abnormalities alter the way the body uses and stores fats, which can cause high blood cholesterol levels, so it is important that they are identified and treated as early as possible.

- Disorders that increase the risk of CHD include diabetes, an underactive thyroid gland and gout.

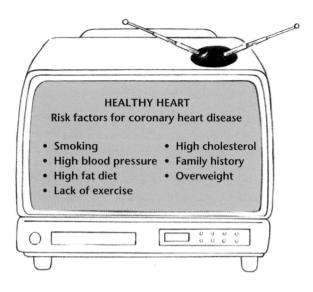

HEALTHY HEART
Risk factors for coronary heart disease

- Smoking
- High blood pressure
- High fat diet
- Lack of exercise
- High cholesterol
- Family history
- Overweight

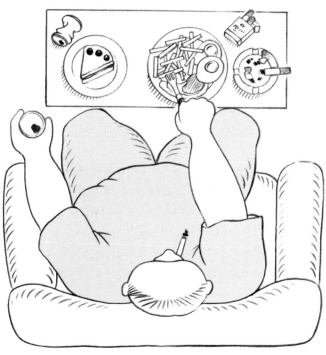

Angina

- Angina is a feeling of pressing tightness or pain across the chest that may spread outwards to the shoulders, upper arms, neck, jaw and even the back. It happens when the heart needs more oxygen than the blood flowing through the coronary arteries can supply, and it is nearly always caused by narrowing of one or more of the arteries as a result of disease.

- Angina of effort occurs with exercise, such as walking uphill, and is worse after a meal and in cold or windy conditions; symptoms usually disappear after 1–2 minutes of rest. Angina also occurs with emotion.

- Angina that occurs more and more frequently, or with less and less exertion over a period of days, weeks or months is called progressive or unstable angina. The pain may begin to start when you are not active and may wake you from sleep. Angina at rest usually means that a coronary artery is becoming increasingly blocked by a fatty deposit (atheromatous plaque) and that a blood clot may also be forming.

- These more serious symptoms mean that urgent investigation and treatment – perhaps with a stay in hospital – are needed to minimize the risk of a heart attack or a disturbance of the heart's normal electrical activity.

- Treatment of angina involves the removal or treatment of risk factors (smoking, high cholesterol or high blood pressure). Aspirin, drugs to slow the heart (beta-blockers) and vasodilators to relax arteries and veins (e.g. glyceryl trinitrate – GTN) are also prescribed. Sometimes procedures to enlarge or bypass coronary artery narrowing are required.

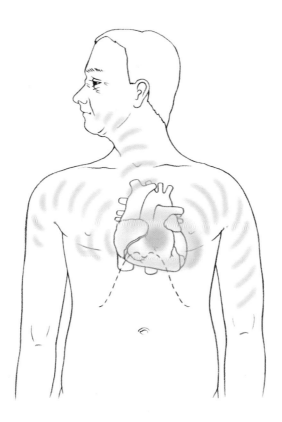

CORONARY ARTERY

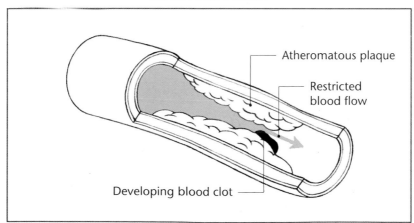

Atheromatous plaque

Restricted
blood flow

Developing blood clot

Heart attack (myocardial infarction)

- Heart attack is known to doctors as myocardial infarction or MI. In an MI, part of the heart muscle dies. This is usually caused by a blood clot (coronary thrombosis), which has formed at the site of a fatty deposit (atheromatous plaque), blocking one of the coronary arteries supplying the heart and depriving the tissues of oxygen. Within minutes of the artery becoming blocked, the muscle starts to die.

- The pain of MI resembles angina in character and is felt in the same places – across the chest and radiating to the shoulders, arms, neck, jaw and back – but is more severe and prolonged, lasting from about 30 minutes to several hours, and is associated with sweating, nausea and vomiting. A patient with an MI may collapse and, without treatment, one out of every eight MI patients will die.

- Emergency admission to hospital and treatment are essential. Modern treatment means that twice as many people survive MI nowadays than 20 years ago.

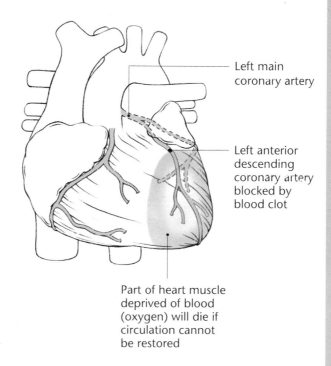

Left main
coronary artery

Left anterior
descending
coronary artery
blocked by
blood clot

Part of heart muscle
deprived of blood
(oxygen) will die if
circulation cannot
be restored

CORONARY ARTERY

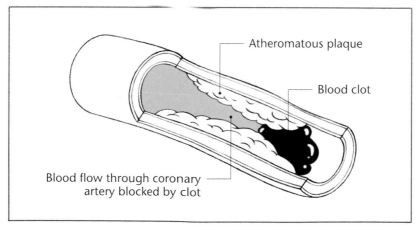

Atheromatous plaque

Blood clot

Blood flow through coronary
artery blocked by clot

Treating heart attack (myocardial infarction)

- Treatment for a myocardial infarction (MI) has three main aims: to relieve pain, to look for and treat any disturbances in the heart's normal electrical activity (usually done in a coronary care unit), and to reopen the blocked artery with drugs or, occasionally, directly using balloons (angioplasty). Drugs used include aspirin and 'clot-busters' such as streptokinase and TPA.

- Other drugs, such as beta-blockers and ACE inhibitors, may be prescribed to help decrease the load on your heart as it heals, and you will probably spend 3–5 days gradually getting mobile again. Any risk factors for coronary heart disease (CHD) – including smoking, high blood cholesterol and high blood pressure – will be investigated and treated at this time.

- Sometimes the first MI is followed by mechanical problems with the heart, anginal pain, or another MI, and these will be investigated and treated quickly.

- After an MI, most patients spend 4–6 weeks at home recovering physically and psychologically. Patients can expect to return to their normal level of activity during that time, and the hospital will probably provide a cardiac rehabilitation programme to help with this.

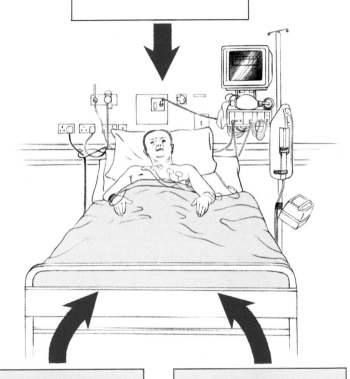

PAIN RELIEF

Morphine
Diamorphine

MONITORING OF THE HEART

Identifies sudden rhythm
changes of the heart
(ventricular fibrillation/
ventricular tachycardia)

TREATMENT

Drugs
- Asprin
- TPA   } 'Clot
- Streptokinase } busters'
- Beta-blockers
- ACE inhibitors

Angioplasty

Heart failure

- Heart failure is a condition with many causes, in which the heart is unable to meet all the demands of the body tissues for oxygen. Although it is a serious condition, heart failure can be effectively treated.

- Heart failure has several causes. The most common causes are damage to the heart muscle by a previous heart attack and high blood pressure. A less common cause of heart failure is narrowing (stenosis) or leaking (regurgitation) of the aortic or mitral valves of the heart.

- The most common symptom of heart failure is fatigue, which may make it an effort to carry out normal daily tasks. In heart failure, the kidneys actively retain more salt and water than usual in the body, which is why the abdomen and legs may become swollen. Breathlessness on exertion and on lying flat may be caused by the lung tissues being swollen with water.

- Most patients will probably need to attend hospital for assessment of their symptoms. However, the good news is that treatment for heart failure is usually very effective.

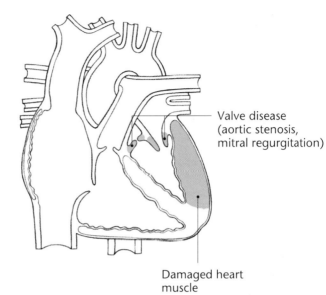

Valve disease
(aortic stenosis,
mitral regurgitation)

Damaged heart
muscle

SYMPTOMS
• Fatigue • Breathlessness (on effort and at night) • Swelling of legs and abdomen

CAUSES	
• Previous heart attack • High blood pressure • Valve disease	• Metabolic diseases • Viruses

Treating heart failure

- Treatment for heart failure is usually very effective. Sometimes the cause of failure can be put right: a defective valve can be replaced, a 'blow-out' (aneurysm) in the heart wall repaired, or the heart's own blood supply improved. The main treatment, however, is with drugs, which have dramatically improved the outlook for people with heart failure in recent years.

- Diuretics relieve swelling and breathlessness caused by water retention, by stimulating the kidneys to get rid of more water and salt in the urine.

- ACE inhibitors are very effective in heart failure. They decrease the work of the heart by relaxing arteries, and by hindering the action of a chemical (Angiotensin Converting Enzyme) that is involved in making the arteries contract. In heart failure, the heart tends to enlarge and become a less efficient pump, but ACE inhibitors help to stop this happening.

- Patients may have to stay in hospital so that drugs to stimulate the heart can be given directly into a vein. Sometimes digoxin is needed to regulate and increase the strength of the heart's pumping action.

- With appropriate treatment, you should be able to live a fairly full and active life with only slight restrictions on physical activity. To achieve this, it is also very important to adopt a healthy 'lifestyle'. The doctor will advise you not to smoke, to keep your weight down, to eat less salt, to exercise gently but regularly, and perhaps to restrict your fluid intake.

DIURETICS

- Amiloride
- Bendrofluazide
- Bumetanide
- Frusemide

ACE INHIBITORS

- Captopril
- Enalapril
- Lisinopril
- Ramipril

CARDIAC GLYCOSIDE

- Digoxin

HEART STIMULANTS

- Adrenaline
- Dopamine
- Dobutamine

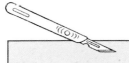

SURGERY

- Valve repair
- Valve replacement
- Aneurysm repair
- Improvements to coronary blood supply

LIFESTYLE

- No smoking
- Lower blood pressure
- Lose weight
- Healthy diet
- Regular exercise
- Reduce salt intake

Hypertension (high blood pressure)

- A diagnosis of hypertension means that the blood pressure is generally higher than it should be. Most people who have hypertension have no symptoms, but if it is not treated, it increases the risk of a stroke, heart attack and kidney problems.

- Blood pressure is measured as part of any examination of the heart and circulation. While the patient is sitting or semi-reclining, a rubber cuff is placed around the upper arm and inflated to compress the artery. The pressure in the cuff is then gradually lowered and the appearance and disappearance of sounds in the artery gives the highest (systolic) and lowest (diastolic) blood pressures, both of which are important to know.

- Blood pressure differs between individuals and varies with activity, time of day and level of stress, so several measurements at different times or over several days, or monitoring with a portable machine, may be needed to find out whether your blood pressure is inappropriately high for you personally.

- Hypertension is not a disease and its cause is usually unknown. However, it can be caused by kidney disease, narrowing of the arteries (e.g. aorta, kidney arteries), and rare hormone abnormalities.

- Drugs to control blood pressure and so diminish these risks include diuretics, artery-relaxing drugs and beta-blockers.

- To keep your blood pressure down to a desirable level, you should not smoke, keep your weight down, eat a balanced diet with no excess salt, and exercise regularly. Any drugs prescribed will probably need to be taken long-term.

Daytime portable blood pressure record in a normal individual shows considerable variation in level

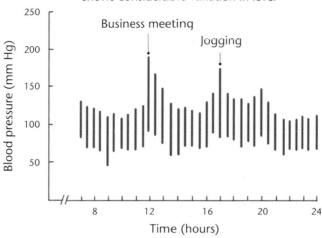

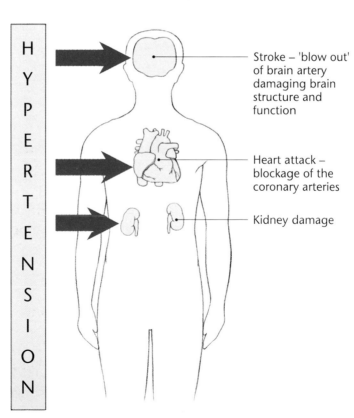

Sudden changes in heart rhythm (arrhythmias)

- An arrhythmia is a disturbance in the rhythm of the heart beat. Palpitations, when you become aware of the beat of your heart, are an extremely common kind of arrhythmia and are usually harmless, but some need investigating.

- In ordinary palpitations, the heart 'skips and jumps', and misses a beat before resetting to normal. Palpitations occur with stress, tiredness or exercise, and after drinking tea, coffee or alcohol.

- Sustained tachycardia (rapid heartbeat) is when the heart unexpectedly starts to beat quickly, in a regular or irregular way, which may last for minutes or even hours. During this time you may sweat, and feel breathless, light-headed and generally unwell.

- Any abnormal tachycardia lasting more than about 20 minutes, or with loss of consciousness, needs investigation. Most regular tachycardias that originate in the heart's upper chambers (supraventricular) are tiresome rather than dangerous.

- Fibrillation (rapid disorganized beating) of the upper heart chambers (atria) is relatively common and usually requires hospital assessment and treatment. Drugs may stop or control this arrhythmia and blood thinning (with aspirin or warfarin) is often helpful.

- Fibrillation of the lower heart chambers (ventricles) causes rapid loss of consciousness, and is fatal unless immediately treated with cardiopulmonary resuscitation ('kiss of life') and electrical 'defibrillation' in which the heart is 'shocked' back into a normal rhythm.

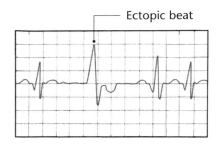

Ectopic beat

ECTOPIC BEAT

- Common
- May be frequent
- Nearly always benign
- Normally comes and goes

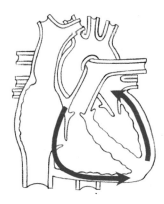

SUPRAVENTRICULAR TACHYCARDIA

Rapid heart beat caused by a wavefront of electricity circling between the upper (atria) and lower (ventricles) chambers of the heart

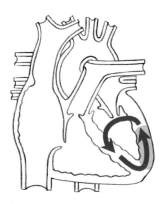

VENTRICULAR TACHYCARDIA

Rapid heart beat caused by a wavefront of electricity circling within the lower chamber (ventricle) of the heart

Bacterial endocarditis

- In endocarditis, bacteria that have entered the bloodstream, usually from the mouth but sometimes from another part of the body, cause an infection of the valves and lining of the heart that is fatal if not treated.

- People whose heart valves do not work correctly or who have other heart abnormalities have an increased risk of developing endocarditis. It is important for them to keep their teeth in good condition with regular dental check-ups, and they should receive antibiotics if their dental work causes any bleeding.

- Endocarditis sometimes comes on suddenly, but usually causes illness for several weeks, with night sweats, weight loss and often aches and pains. Occasionally, an abscess (in which pus collects) can form in the heart, or part of an infected valve may be carried away in the blood and block the circulation in another organ, causing a stroke or other complications.

- Patients need to go to hospital so that the bacteria responsible for the infection can be identified. Antibiotics to kill the bacteria have to be given direct into a vein close to the heart for 4–6 weeks. If the infection causes serious damage to a heart valve, an operation to fit a new valve may be necessary.

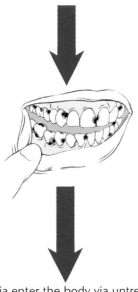

RISK FACTORS

- Pre-existing valve abnormalities
- Bad teeth

Bacteria enter the body via untreated tooth decay and are carried by the blood to the heart

EFFECTS

- Chronic illness
- Fevers/sweats
- Weight loss
- Bacteria in blood

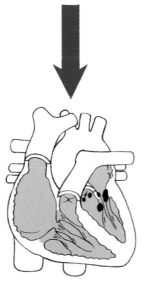

TREATMENT

- Admission to hospital
- Prolonged antibiotic therapy
- Occasionally, heart valve surgery

Congenital heart disease

- Congenital diseases are problems that people are born with. The most common problems in congenital heart disease are either extra holes between parts of the heart or the main arteries so that oxygenated (red) blood mixes with deoxygenated (blue) blood, or narrowing of an artery, heart chamber, or heart valve so that blood flow is restricted. Both types of abnormality can be present together.

- Most such defects give no trouble, though some – particularly the more complex kinds – can seriously reduce the amount of oxygen in the blood that is pumped round the body, so that the patient's skin looks blue (cyanotic).

- Minor heart defects, such as a small hole between the two ventricles, may not need repairing and may even heal themselves. Most of the more serious congenital defects can be repaired by surgery.

- Most people with congenital heart disease lead full and active lives, but may need regular or infrequent hospital check-ups.

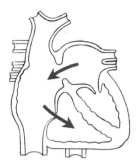

ATRIAL SEPTAL DEFECT

- Hole between the two upper chambers
- Blood passes from the left to right atrium and into the lungs
- Excess blood recirculates through the lungs

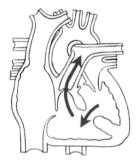

VENTRICULAR SEPTAL DEFECT

- Hole between the two main pump chambers
- Blood passes from the left to right ventricle
- Excess blood recirculates through the lungs
- Large holes can flood or damage the lungs
- Small holes cause no problems

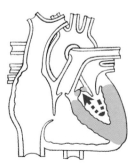

AORTIC STENOSIS

- Strain on the left ventricle pumping blood to the body
- Can damage the left ventricle
- May need surgery

Blackouts

- A blackout is loss of consciousness that may or may not be related to the heart.

- An abrupt speeding up or slowing down of the heart rhythm can cause a blackout with little or no warning, so that the individual suddenly drops to the ground and may be hurt in falling. The patient looks pale and lifeless, but soon recovers and can immediately remember what has happened.

- This kind of blackout needs hospital investigation. Some patients will be given a heart pacemaker, while others will receive treatment with drugs.

- Simple faints do not need investigation unless they happen very often. They can be associated with illness, standing for a long time, fear, excessive heat or tiredness, prolonged coughing, and many other things. Older men may blackout briefly after passing urine, and standing up suddenly after sitting can cause light-headedness.

- Before a faint, a person may become very pale, sweat, yawn, and have a buzzing sound in the ears. The best way to avoid losing consciousness is to lie down flat – the floor is safest – preferably with the legs in the air!

- Other causes of blackouts unrelated to the heart include epilepsy, stroke, drugs and low blood sugar.

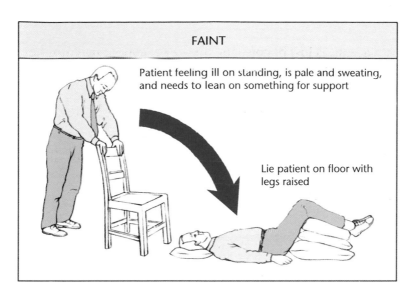

FAINT

Patient feeling ill on standing, is pale and sweating, and needs to lean on something for support

Lie patient on floor with legs raised

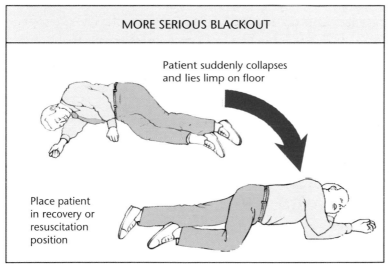

MORE SERIOUS BLACKOUT

Patient suddenly collapses and lies limp on floor

Place patient in recovery or resuscitation position

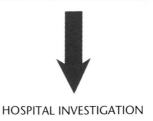

HOSPITAL INVESTIGATION

Treating heart disorders with drugs

- Many different types of drugs have been developed to help patients with heart disorders. Each type acts in a particular way on the heart, arteries or other organs.

- Many of these drugs not only reduce symptoms, but also avoid complications developing, and so help the patient to live longer.

- The main types of drugs used to treat heart disorders are beta-blockers, diuretics, aspirin, ACE inhibitors, digoxin, HMG CoA reductase inhibitors, vasodilators and calcium antagonists.

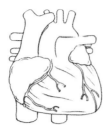

HEART	
Drug	*When given*
Beta-blockers	Heart attack, hypertension
ACE inhibitors	Heart attack, hypertension
Digoxin	Atrial fibrillation
Vasodilators	Angina
Amiodarone	Serious arrhythmias

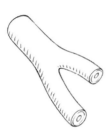

ARTERIES	
Drug	*When given*
Aspirin	Narrowing of the arteries
ACE inhibitors	Hypertension, heart failure
Calcium antagonists	Hypertension, angina

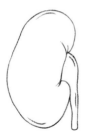

KIDNEYS	
Drug	*When given*
Diuretics	Hypertension, heart failure
ACE inhibitors	Heart failure

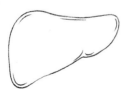

LIVER	
Drug	*When given*
HMG CoA reductase inhibitors	High cholesterol

Drugs used for heart disorders

- ACE inhibitors help increase the flow of blood through arteries by hindering the formation of a natural chemical in the body that makes them contract. They are useful for treating high blood pressure, heart failure and heart attack.

- Aspirin inhibits blood clotting and is given to patients with any heart or circulation condition in which blood clots form (e.g. heart attack or stroke).

- Beta-blockers slow down the heart rate and may be given to patients with high blood pressure or angina, or those recovering from a heart attack.

- Calcium antagonists improve blood flow by relaxing the arteries, and some also slow the heart. They are used in patients with high blood pressure and angina.

- Digoxin strengthens and slows the heart's pumping action; it is used to treat heart failure and atrial fibrillation, which is a rapid, disorganized contraction of the upper heart chambers.

- Diuretics stimulate the kidneys to excrete more salt and water in the urine in patients with high blood pressure or heart failure.

- HMG CoA reductase inhibitors reduce cholesterol production by the liver, and lower blood cholesterol in patients with heart disease or at particular risk from high blood cholesterol.

- Vasodilators reduce the amount of oxygen that the heart needs and are often given to patients with angina.

TYPE OF DRUG	EXAMPLES
ACE inhibitors	Captopril Enalapril Lisinopril Ramipril
Aspirin	
Beta-blockers	Atenolol Bisoprolol Metoprolol
Calcium antagonists	Diltiazem Nifedipine Verapamil
Digoxin	
Diuretics	Amiloride Bendrofluazide Frusemide
HMG CoA reductase inhibitors	Lovastatin Simvastatin
Vasodilators	Glyceryl trinitrate (GTN) Isosorbide mononitrate Nicorandil

Hospital visits for heart disorders

- People who visit their doctor with symptoms that could be caused by heart or circulation trouble may be referred to a hospital outpatient clinic to be examined by a consultant cardiologist. Before your hospital visit, your family doctor will contact the specialist with information about your symptoms.

- Possible heart symptoms could be chest pain, unusual breathlessness, palpitations that go on for a long time, some kinds of blackout or an unusual heart sound (murmur).

- On your first visit to the hospital, preliminary investigations, such as an electrocardiogram (ECG) or heart monitoring, may be carried out.

- You may be asked to attend the hospital fasting, that is having had no food or drink since the previous night. At the hospital, there is usually a reception desk and waiting area where the nurse or assistant will show you where to go for any preliminary investigations and you may be asked for a urine sample.

- Many patients need only one hospital visit, but you may be invited back for further tests. These could include exercise testing, heart scanning or monitoring of ECG or blood pressure.

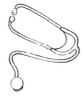

Patient with possible heart
symptoms sees family doctor

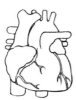

Family doctor refers patient to consultant
cardiologist at hospital

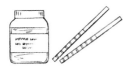
Out Patients

Hospital invites patient to attend
outpatient clinic

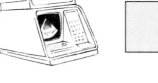

Patient attends hospital fasting, bringing
urine sample, has preliminary ECG
and sees the specialist

Specialist may ask for further tests

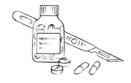

Specialist makes diagnosis and
recommends treatment

Examining the eyes

- An eye examination gives the hospital cardiologist clues as to the state of your circulation, showing up any fatty deposits, bleeding in the light-sensitive retina at the back of the eye, and changes associated with diabetes, high blood pressure or other conditions.

- By shining a focused bright light from an instrument called an ophthalmoscope into the eye, the cardiologist can directly inspect the retina, the small arteries and veins that run over it, and the optic nerve that carries impulses from the eye to the brain.

- Usually both eyes will be examined. You may see colours differently for a few minutes after having the bright light shone into your eyes, but this is quite normal.

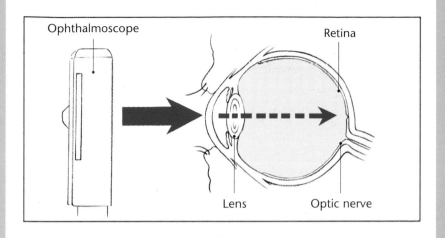

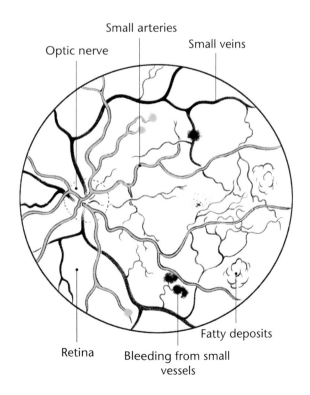

Testing the urine

- Urine analysis is a very important early screening test. Several substances that give clues to the presence of various medical conditions can be simply detected by dipping specially treated 'dipsticks' into the urine.

- The most important substances that can be detected by 'dipsticks' are sugar (glucose) which may indicate diabetes, excessive protein which is associated with kidney malfunction or infection, and other substances which point to liver disease.

- A sample of your urine will probably be routinely tested when you visit the hospital outpatient clinic. It can also be sent to a laboratory to be checked for infection and for any cells and sediment to be examined under the microscope. Sometimes all the urine you pass in a 24-hour period will be collected so that the protein content and other substances produced by the body can be analysed more easily.

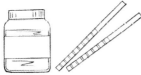

- Urine analysis
- Chemical identified by 'dipstick' in urine sample

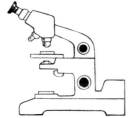

- Diabetes
- Kidney malfunction
- Liver diseases

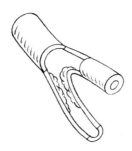

- Urine examined in the laboratory for infection, cells or sediment

- Diabetes is associated with narrowing of the coronary arteries
- Kidney inflammation is associated with endocarditis and high blood pressure

The electrocardiogram (ECG)

- The ECG is a simple, painless and common investigation which takes only a few minutes. It gives the hospital cardiologist useful information about many aspects of the heart's performance, including disturbances of rhythm (arrhythmias), heart attacks and thickening (hypertrophy) of the heart muscle.

- During the ECG, the electrical activity of the heart is picked up by electrodes attached to the skin and displayed as a line on a screen or paper chart. Usually six electrodes are placed on the chest and one electrode on each arm and on each leg.

- Sometimes your heart rhythm needs to be recorded over 24 hours to detect arrhythmias that do not happen all the time. In this case, four or five leads from electrodes on your chest will be connected to a recorder that is usually worn on a waist belt. The recording is then analysed by a computer (the 24-hour ECG contains so much information that a computer takes up to half an hour to analyse it!).

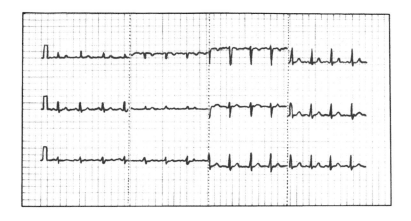

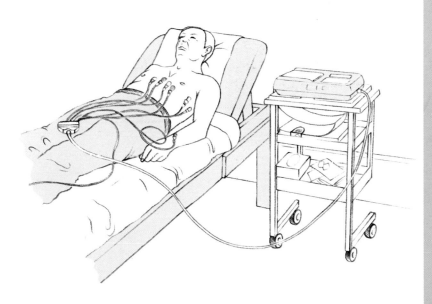

The chest X-ray

- An X-ray picture (radiograph) of the chest is useful for detecting lung disorders, and also helps the cardiologist to spot signs of heart disease.

- The radiograph can show up any enlargement of the whole heart and some of its chambers. It can also show congestion of the lungs, in which there is a build-up of fluid causing breathlessness and which may be a consequence of heart disease.

- The chest X-ray is carried out in the hospital's radiology department. You will probably be asked to stand or sit in front of the X-ray plate, and breathe in and hold your breath for a few seconds (so as not to blur the image) while the radiographer takes the picture.

- The dose of X-rays needed to make the radiograph is extremely small.

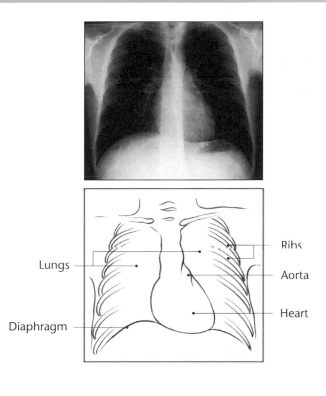

Lungs

Ribs

Aorta

Heart

Diaphragm

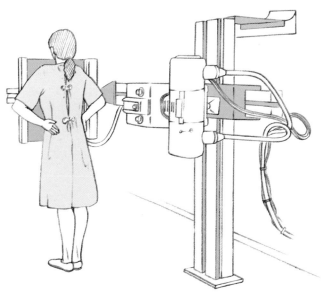

Visualizing the heart by ultrasound

- Cardiac ultrasound is a straightforward but very useful test on the heart. It measures heart size, the function of the heart valves and chambers, and how well the heart is performing.

- Cardiac ultrasound is painless and has revolutionized the assessment of many heart conditions over the last decade. There are no specific risks associated with the procedure.

- It is usually performed in a darkened room (to enable the monitor to be seen more easily) using a probe with special ultrasound jelly on the chest. The ultrasound 'beam' has a very high frequency that is inaudible.

- The test takes about 10–15 minutes. You may be asked to lie in a particular position to avoid air from the lungs interfering with the picture.

- Doppler ultrasound is used to measure the flow of the blood within the heart. It is particularly useful in assessing leakage and narrowing of the heart valves (e.g. aortic stenosis, mitral stenosis, aortic regurgitation, mitral regurgitation), and for assessing shunts (holes) within the heart.

- Occasionally, it can be useful to examine the heart from behind. This can be done using a special ultrasound probe that is swallowed. This technique, which is called transoesophageal ultrasound, is usually carried out as a day-case procedure under light sedation.

ULTRASOUND SCAN

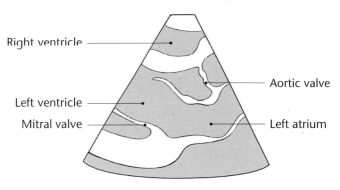

Right ventricle

Aortic valve

Left ventricle

Mitral valve

Left atrium

DOPPLER SIGNAL FROM A DISEASED AORTIC VALVE

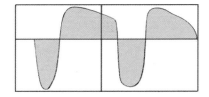

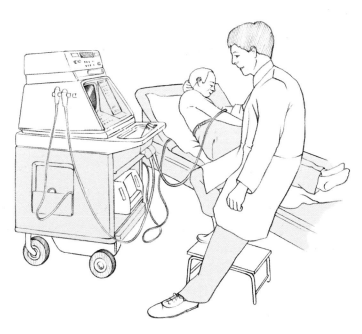

The exercise ECG

- Exercise ECG testing (sometimes called treadmill testing) is helpful where angina is suspected or to assess the severity of heart disease (e.g. after a heart attack).

- Treadmill testing during the early recovery phase after a heart attack often involves low levels of exercise, but more commonly a 'symptom-limited' test is performed. This involves walking on a moving pavement (the treadmill) or a bicycle at a series of standard speeds and inclines. These start at low level and increase, usually at 3-minute intervals.

- The test looks at symptoms, blood pressure, exercise ability and changes in the electrical heart recording (the electrocardiogram or ECG) during and after exercise. Chest pain, undue breathlessness or fatigue or significant changes in blood pressure, heart rate or the ECG would all lead to the test being stopped.

- A trained technician and, sometimes, a doctor will be in attendance throughout. Monitoring of the ECG is routine for several minutes after the exercise phase of the test is over.

- Avoid a heavy meal before an exercise test, and wear comfortable clothing and shoes suitable for walking.

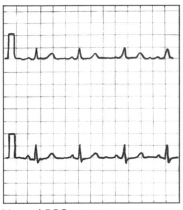

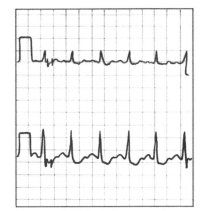

Normal ECG at rest

Abnormal ECG during exercise

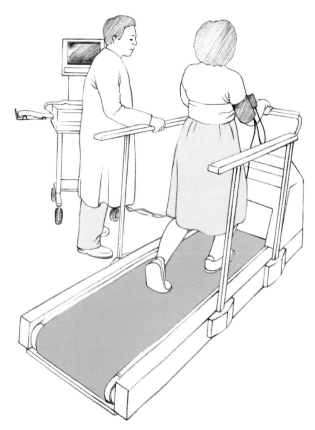

Cardiac catheterization (angiogram)

- Cardiac catheterization can be carried out on a day patient or inpatient basis, and is mainly used to assess the site and severity of narrowing of the coronary arteries in detail. It is occasionally necessary to study the function of the heart valves, the heart pump or other heart defects.

- A routine medical examination will be conducted before the test and some blood samples may be taken. The catheterization laboratory is staffed by nurses and technicians under the direction of the cardiologist, and houses the highly sophisticated equipment necessary to conduct the test efficiently and safely.

- Under local anaesthesia (often with a light sedative), a fine tube is inserted into the heart through a blood vessel either in the groin (femoral) or arm (brachial), or occasionally through a neck vein. You will be asked to take a deep breath and hold it as the dye is injected to enable the arteries to be seen. A hot flushing sensation often occurs after the dye is injected into the main heart pump (the left ventricle). Multiple pictures of the coronary arteries are usually obtained. A routine coronary angiogram takes about 30–40 minutes.

- After the procedure, bed-rest for 4–6 hours is usual. Some bruising and discomfort at the site of tube insertion is common for 1–2 days, and vigorous exercise and driving should be avoided for 48 hours.

- Most people comment, after cardiac catheterization, that the procedure was much less unpleasant than they had anticipated and that it was thinking about it that was the worse aspect!

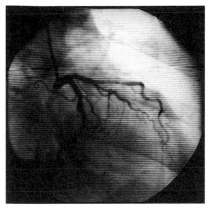

X-ray picture of coronary artery
obtained during cardiac catheterization

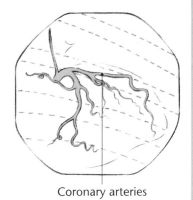

Coronary arteries

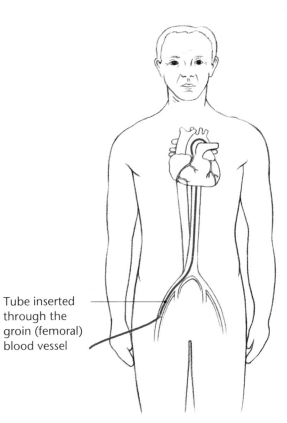

Tube inserted
through the
groin (femoral)
blood vessel

Coronary angioplasty

- Coronary angioplasty involves inserting a balloon into a diseased (blocked/narrowed) coronary artery through an artery in the groin or arm. Inflation of the balloon across the area of narrowing 'squashes' the deposit causing the narrowing and flattens it against the wall of the artery. On removal of the balloon, normal blood flow is restored.

- Sometimes it is necessary to implant a metal scaffold or stent within the artery to keep it open.

- The procedure is performed in the cardiac catheterization laboratory. A local anaesthetic and appropriate sedation are used along with the drugs to stop blood clotting (aspirin, heparin and sometimes warfarin) and to relax the coronary arteries (glyceryl trinitrate).

- It is usual to stay in hospital for 1–3 days and to have a few days of convalescence after discharge home.

- Very rarely (1% of cases), the artery may be damaged by the balloon. If, as a result, there is a risk of heart attack, then an emergency heart bypass operation may be necessary. A more common (but less serious) problem is re-narrowing of the artery after successful enlargement. This happens in 20–25% of individuals and a second angioplasty or the insertion of a stent may be required to reduce the risk of recurrence.

- Coronary angioplasty has advantages over coronary surgery in that it involves a shorter period of time in hospital and recovery is quicker. However, some patients with complicated narrowings or blockages, or those with several coronary arteries affected, are best treated by a coronary bypass operation.

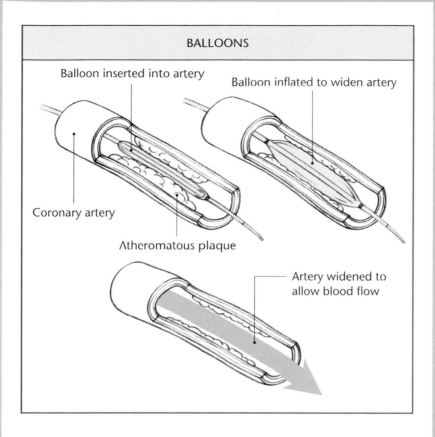

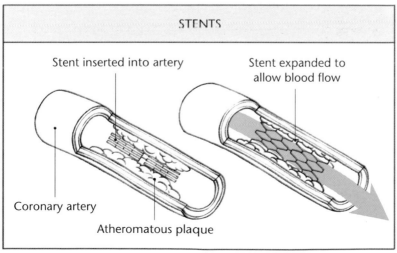

Heart pacemakers

- The electrical activity of the upper chamber of the heart (the atrium) or the conduction of electricity through the heart from atrium to the lower chamber (ventricle) may fail partially or completely. This can cause or threaten unconsciousness or sudden severe light-headedness.

- The condition may be temporary (for example after a heart attack) and the pacemaker is therefore only required for a matter of days. For many the pacemaker is required lifelong.

- With a temporary pacemaker, a wire is usually inserted through an arm or neck vein into the right ventricle and connected to an external pacemaker box. Permanent pacemakers are much smaller and are implanted under the skin (usually below the collar bone) in an operating theatre and often under local anaesthesia with sedation. The procedure usually takes less than 1 hour. Pacemaker implantation is one of the most successful and straightforward procedures in cardiology today.

- Permanent pacemakers are highly sophisticated and can be attached to the upper or lower chambers of the heart, or both as required. They are highly reliable and last many years. Many centres will allow patients to go home on the same day or the day after implantation (provided the pacemaker unit and the X-ray check are satisfactory). A check-up after 1 month and annually thereafter is necessary. Some wound discomfort and some bruising for a few days is usual. Stitches may need to be removed after 5–8 days.

- Patients are not allowed to drive for the first month after permanent pacemaker implantation.

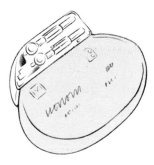

Permanent pacemaker

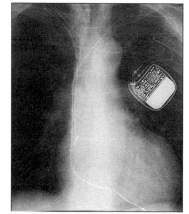

X-ray showing the position of the pacemaker and the wires to the heart

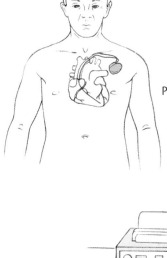

Permanent pacemaker

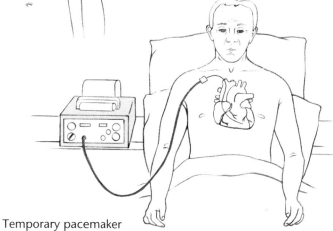

Temporary pacemaker

Specialist electrical treatment

- Over the last few years, it has been possible to use special radiofrequency current to provide heat to destroy the abnormal pathways within the heart that are responsible for certain forms of heart rhythm disturbance. This type of treatment is called an ablation procedure.

- This type of treatment is particularly suitable for rhythm disturbances associated with abnormal electrical conduction between the atrium and ventricle – either extra connections away from the normal conduction system (e.g. the Wolff-Parkinson-White Syndrome) or with double cables within the normal heart conduction system (called AV nodal re-entry).

- Using local anaesthesia, wires are placed precisely within the heart to locate the extra pathways involved and these are destroyed by the radiofrequency ablation catheter using heat. X-rays are used to ensure that the wire is in the correct position. The procedure can take some hours to complete and it is usual for patients to spend 2 days in hospital.

- This type of procedure has the great advantage, if completely successful (as is usual), of avoiding the need for long-term drug treatment. It is best suited to those who have recurrent episodes of an abnormal fast heart rhythm or those in whom drug treatment has not proved particularly successful or has significant side-effects.

- Referral to a specialist heart centre with this expertise is essential. Treatment of some other types of electrical disturbance of heart rhythm is also possible.

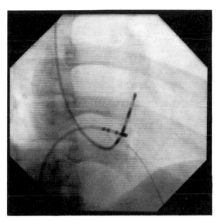

28

X-ray showing the position of the wires
during the ablation procedure

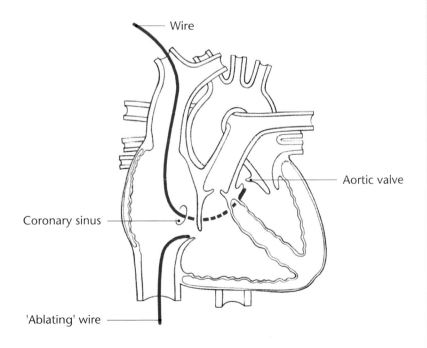

Wire

Aortic valve

Coronary sinus

'Ablating' wire

Cardioversion

- Certain types of disturbance of heart rhythm can be corrected by passing a high voltage electric charge through the heart. This procedure is called cardioversion.

- Paddles are usually applied externally (one to the front of the chest and one to the left side) to deliver between 50 and 300 joules of electrical power to 'shock' the heart back to its normal rhythm.

- Cardioversion is usually undertaken under general anaesthesia or, in an emergency, using heavy sedation. It takes a matter of minutes.

- Patients with rhythm disturbances affecting the upper chambers of the heart (the atria) undergoing cardioversion often receive warfarin for some weeks before the procedure. This is to minimize the risk of blood clot formation within the atria and subsequent dislodgement of the clot causing a stroke. Warfarin is usually continued for some weeks after a successful procedure. Cardioversion can be repeated if necessary.

- Very occasionally, patients with recurring life-threatening rhythm disturbances require insertion of an implantable cardioverter defibrillator. This sophisticated and expensive device will recognize life-threatening rhythm disturbances and treat them appropriately, if necessary by delivering a cardioversion electrical charge similar to that used with the external defibrillator. These devices are relatively new. Several days in hospital is usual and implantation involves a general anaesthetic.

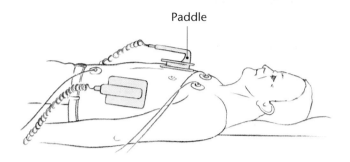

29

Paddle

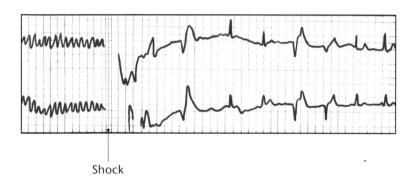

Shock

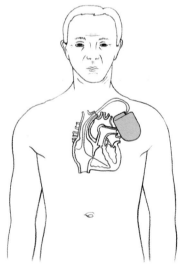

Implantable
cardioverter
defibrillator

Mail Order

Additional copies of this book and other titles in the *Patient Pictures* series are available at a unit price of £10.95 (post-paid in the UK only).

Current titles include:
- Cardiology
- Fertility and infertility
- Gastroenterology
- Gynaecology
- Prostatic diseases and treatments
- Respiratory diseases
- Rheumatology
- Urological surgery

Please send your name and address, quantity required, and a cheque for the appropriate amount made payable to 'Health Press' to:

Health Press
Elizabeth House
Queen Street
Abingdon
Oxford OX14 3JR

Health Press titles are available at special discounts when purchased in bulk quantities for trusts, associations or institutions. Please call our Special Sales Department in Abingdon on:

Tel: 01235 523233
Fax: 01235 523238